Anti infla
Foods Chart

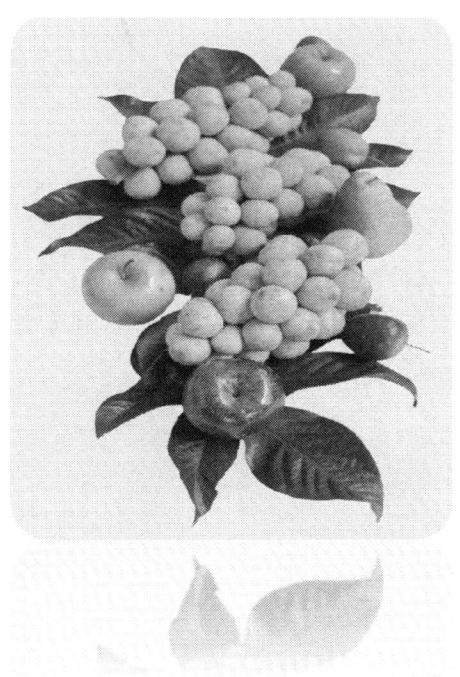

What to Eat While on an Anti-Inflammatory Diet: anti-inflammatory food list chart (A No-Stress Meal Plan with 30 Easy Recipes to simplify your healing)

Zeerah Amelia

Copyright © 2023 by Zeerah Amelia

All rights reserved. No part of this book may be reproduced, stored in a retrieval system, or transmitted in any form or by any means, electronic, mechanical, photocopying, recording, or otherwise, without prior written permission from the publisher.

<u>Disclaimer Notice:</u> Please note the information contained within this document is for educational and entertainment purposes only. Under no circumstances will any blame or legal responsibility be held against the publisher, or author, for any damages, reparation, or+ monetary loss due to the information contained within this book, either directly or indirectly.

All effort has been executed to present accurate, up-to-date, reliable, and complete information. No warranties of any kind are declared or implied.

TABLE OF CONTENTS

INTRODUCTION 7

GETTING STARTED 9

ANTI INFLAMMATORY FOODS CHART:
CATEGORIZING FOOD GROUPS FOR EASY REFERENCE 11

- Fresh Fruit 11
- Dried Fruit 17
- Vegetables 22
- Plant-Based Proteins 28
- Fatty Fish 30
- Whole Grains 36
- Leafy Greens: 41
- Herbs & Spices 45
- Nuts & Seeds 51
- Foods Filled With Omega-3 Fatty Acids 56
- Coffee 60
- Green Tea 63
- Dark Chocolate (In Moderation) 66
- Red Wine (In Moderation) 68

ANTI INFLAMMATORY DIET MEAL PLANNING TIPS: 73

QUICK AND EASY ANTI-INFLAMMATORY DELICIOUS RECIPES .. 75

BREAKFAST 75
- Avocado and Salmon Breakfast Wrap: 75
- Berry and Almond Smoothie Bowl: 75
- Turmeric Scrambled Eggs: 75
- Greek Yogurt Parfait with Nuts: 76
- Quinoa Breakfast Bowl: 76

LUNCH 76
- Grilled Chicken and Vegetable Salad: 76
- Quinoa and Black Bean Bowl: 77
- Salmon and Sweet Potato Skewers: 77
- Lentil and Vegetable Soup: 77
- Spinach and Chickpea Salad: 78

DINNER: 78
- Baked Turmeric Cod with Quinoa: 78
- Vegetable Stir-Fry with Tofu: 78
- Butternut Squash and Chickpea Curry: 79
- Turkey and Quinoa Stuffed Bell Peppers: 79
- Sweet Potato and Kale Hash: 79

SNACKS 80
- Greek Yogurt with Berries: 80
- Almond Butter and Banana Slices: 80
- Hummus and Veggie Sticks: 80

- Trail Mix with Nuts and Seeds: 80
- Avocado and Tomato on Whole Grain Toast: 81

DESSERTS 81

- Chia Seed Pudding with Berries: 81
- Baked Apples with Cinnamon and Walnuts: 81
- Dark Chocolate and Berry Parfait: 82
- Mango and Coconut Sorbet: 82
- Almond Flour Banana Muffins: 82

SMOOTHIES 83

- Green Detox Smoothie: 83
- Berry Protein Smoothie: 83
- Tropical Turmeric Smoothie: 83
- Avocado and Kale Smoothie: 84
- Chocolate Peanut Butter Banana Smoothie: 84

BUILDING A HEART-HEALTHY FRIENDLY PANTRY: ESSENTIAL GROCERY LIST 85

BREAKFAST 85

CONCLUSION 95

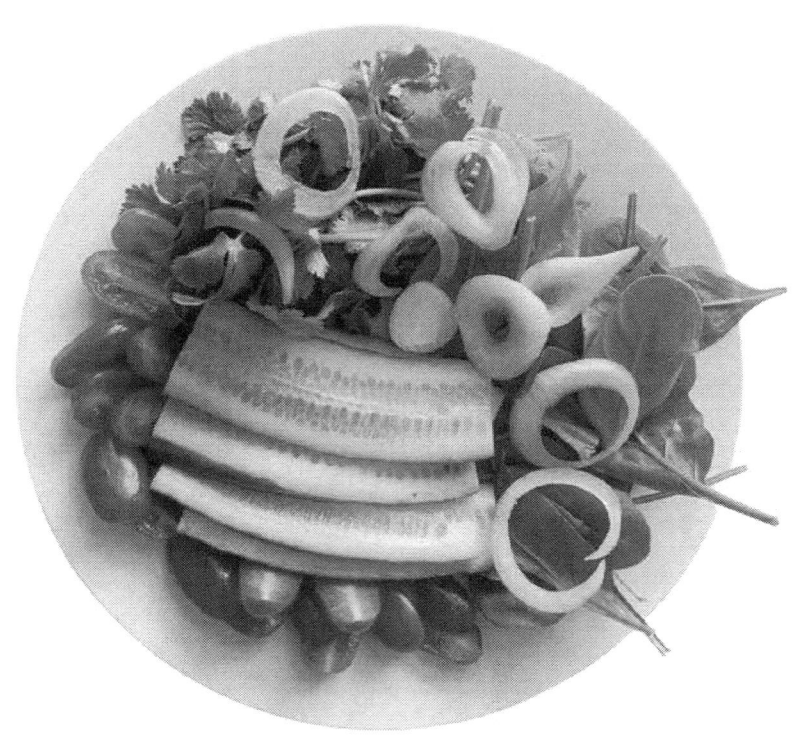

INTRODUCTION

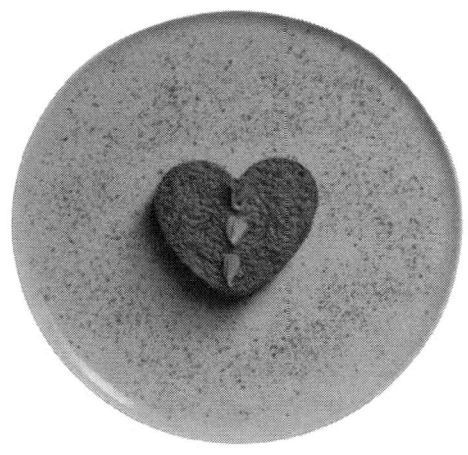

The anti-inflammatory diet is a way of eating that focuses on foods known to reduce inflammation in the body, promoting heart health. Inflammation is linked to various health issues, and this diet aims to combat it.

It involves consuming whole, nutrient-rich foods like fruits, vegetables, nuts, and fatty fish, while minimizing processed foods, sugary drinks, and excessive red meat.

The goal is to promote overall health and potentially alleviate conditions associated with inflammation, such as arthritis or heart disease. By incorporating anti-inflammatory foods, you provide your body with essential nutrients and antioxidants that can help manage inflammation.

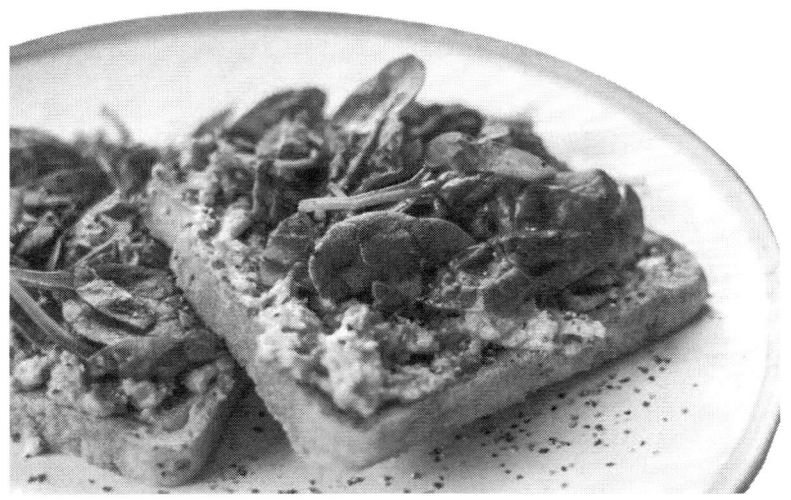

GETTING STARTED

Are you tired of searching for the right foods to support your Anti-inflammatory diet? Do you feel overwhelmed by numerous choices and unsure of how to make the most of your meals? Your search ends here, because the ultimate solution is here

"Anti-inflammatory Foods Chart: Your Essential Guide to What Food to Eat while on Anti-inflammatory Diet, Approved comfort foods to Combat diseases, Increase Your Energy and promote longevity."

Whether you're following popular Heart-Healthy diets like Mediterranean diet, DASH Diet, Whole30 Diet, Plant-Based Diet, Paleo Diet, Gluten-Free Diet, this comprehensive food guide is your go-to resource. We understand the pains and challenges of following Anti-inflammatory diet, and we're here to make it easier for you.

Inside this book, you'll find an extensive list of Anti-inflammatory foods, carefully organized by a food group,

Doctors-Developed, Patient-proven. Each food comes with its Nutritional value per serving, ensuring you can track your intake accurately. Say goodbye to the guesswork and confusion!

But that's not all – we go the extra mile by providing 30 healthy, mouthwatering, Easy to prepare and budget-friendly recipes tailored to the "Anti-inflammatory Diet" with ingredients available in most local grocery stores, specifically designed to satisfy your special taste buds while keeping you on track.

Additionally, our meal prep tips and strategies will help you save time and effortlessly incorporate an Anti-inflammatory meal into your busy schedule. Now If you're ready to take control of your nutrition and experience the transformative power of an Anti-inflammatory diet, "Anti Inflammatory Foods Chart" is your

trusted companion.

Let's embark on this journey together and unlock a healthier, more vibrant you.

ANTI INFLAMMATORY FOODS CHART: CATEGORIZING FOOD GROUPS FOR EASY REFERENCE

- **FRESH FRUIT**

1. Blueberries:

Serving: 1 cup

- *Calories:* ~84
- *Carbs:* 21g
- *Fiber:* 4g

2. Strawberries:

Serving: 1 cup, sliced

- *Calories:* ~50
- *Carbs:* 11g
- *Fiber:* 3g

3. Pineapple:

Serving: **1 cup, diced**

- *Calories:* ~82

- *Carbs:* 22g
- *Fiber:* 2.3g

4. Mango:
Serving: 1 cup, sliced
- *Calories:* ~107
- *Carbs:* 28g
- *Fiber:* 3g

5. Cherries:
Serving: 1 cup
- *Calories:* ~87
- *Carbs:* 22g
- *Fiber:* 3g

6. Papaya:
Serving: 1 cup, cubes
- *Calories:* ~60
- *Carbs:* 15g
- *Fiber:* 3g

7. Oranges:
Serving: 1 medium

- *Calories:* ~62
- *Carbs:* 15g
- *Fiber:* 3g

8. Apples:
Serving: **1 medium**
- *Calories:* ~95
- *Carbs:* 25g
- *Fiber:* 4g

9. Kiwi:
Serving: **2 medium**
- *Calories:* ~93
- *Carbs:* 19g
- *Fiber:* 5g

10. Watermelon:
Serving: **1 cup, diced**
- *Calories:* ~46
- *Carbs:* 11g
- *Fiber:* 1g

11. Grapes:
Serving: **1 cup**
- *Calories:* ~104
- *Carbs:* 27g
- *Fiber:* 1g

12. Raspberries:
Serving: **1 cup**
- *Calories:* ~65
- *Carbs:* 15g
- *Fiber:* 8g

13. Cantaloupe:
Serving: **1 cup, diced**
- *Calories:* ~54
- *Carbs:* 13g
- *Fiber:* 1.5g

14. Grapefruit:
Serving: **1 medium**
- *Calories:* ~52
- *Carbs:* 13g

- *Fiber:* 2g

15. Pomegranate:
***Serving:* 1 cup, arils**

- *Calories:* ~83
- *Carbs:* 19g
- *Fiber:* 4g

16. Cranberries:
***Serving:* 1 cup, whole**

- *Calories:* ~46
- *Carbs:* 12g
- *Fiber:* 4.6g

17. Apricots:
***Serving:* 1 cup, halves**

- *Calories:* ~74
- *Carbs:* 18g
- *Fiber:* 3.3g

18. Bananas:
Serving: **1 medium**
- *Calories:* ~105
- *Carbs:* 27g
- *Fiber:* 3.1g

19. Plums:
Serving: **2 medium**
- *Calories:* ~70
- *Carbs:* 18g
- *Fiber:* 2.3g

20. Peaches:
Serving: **1 medium**
- *Calories:* ~58
- *Carbs:* 15g
- *Fiber:* 2.3g

■ DRIED FRUIT

1. Dried Blueberries:
Serving: 1/4 cup

- *Calories:* ~85
- *Carbs:* 22g
- *Fiber:* 2g

2. Dried Strawberries:
Serving: 1/4 cup

- *Calories:* ~100
- *Carbs:* 25g
- *Fiber:* 3g

3. Dried Pineapple:
Serving: 1/4 cup

- *Calories:* ~96
- *Carbs:* 25g
- *Fiber:* 2.5g

4. Dried Mango:
Serving: 1/4 cup

- *Calories:* ~100

- *Carbs:* 25g
- *Fiber:* 2g

5. Dried Cherries:
Serving: **1/4 cup**
- *Calories:* ~104
- *Carbs:* 26g
- *Fiber:* 2g

6. Dried Papaya:
Serving: **1/4 cup**
- *Calories:* ~59
- *Carbs:* 15g
- *Fiber:* 1g

7. Dried Oranges:
Serving: **1/4 cup**
- *Calories:* ~90
- *Carbs:* 22g
- *Fiber:* 4g

8. Dried Apples:
Serving: **1/4 cup**

- *Calories:* ~104
- *Carbs:* 28g
- *Fiber:* 4g

9. Dried Kiwi:
Serving: 1/4 cup
- *Calories:* ~87
- *Carbs:* 22g
- *Fiber:* 3g

10. Dried Watermelon:
Serving: 1/4 cup
- *Calories:* ~110
- *Carbs:* 29g
- *Fiber:* 3g

11. Raisins:
Serving: 1/4 cup
- *Calories:* ~108
- *Carbs:* 28g
- *Fiber:* 1g

12. Dried Cranberries:
Serving: **1/4 cup**
- *Calories:* ~93
- *Carbs:* 25g
- *Fiber:* 2g

13. Dried Apricots:
Serving: **4 halves**
- *Calories:* ~100
- *Carbs:* 25g
- *Fiber:* 3g

14. Dried Plums (Prunes):
Serving: **5 prunes**
- *Calories:* ~100
- *Carbs:* 26g
- *Fiber:* 3g

15. Dried Grapefruit:
Serving: **1/4 cup**
- *Calories:* ~97
- *Carbs:* 25g

- *Fiber:* 3g

16. Dried Pomegranate Seeds:
Serving: **1/4 cup**

- *Calories:* ~110
- *Carbs:* 26g
- *Fiber:* 5g

17. Dried Cranraisins:
Serving: **1/4 cup**

- *Calories:* ~93
- *Carbs:* 25g
- *Fiber:* 2g

18. Dried Banana Chips:
Serving: **1/4 cup**

- *Calories:* ~100
- *Carbs:* 27g
- *Fiber:* 2g

19. Dried Plum Chips:
Serving: **1/4 cup**

- *Calories:* ~110

- *Carbs:* 26g
- *Fiber:* 3g

20. Dried Peach Slices:
Serving: **1/4 cup**
- *Calories:* ~96
- *Carbs:* 25g
- *Fiber:* 2g

■ VEGETABLES

1. Spinach:
Serving: **1 cup (raw)**
- *Calories:* ~7
- *Carbs:* 1g
- *Fiber:* 0.7g

2. Broccoli:
Serving: **1 cup (chopped)**
- *Calories:* ~55
- *Carbs:* 11g
- *Fiber:* 5g

3. Carrots:
Serving: **1 medium carrot**
- *Calories:* ~25
- *Carbs:* 6g
- *Fiber:* 2g

4. Bell Peppers (Red):
Serving: **1 cup (sliced)**
- *Calories:* ~46
- *Carbs:* 9g
- *Fiber:* 3g

5. Tomatoes:
Serving: **1 medium tomato**
- *Calories:* ~22
- *Carbs:* 5g
- *Fiber:* 2g

6. Cucumbers:
Serving: **1/2 medium cucumber**
- *Calories:* ~23
- *Carbs:* 4g

- *Fiber:* 1g

7. Kale:
Serving: **1 cup (chopped)**
- *Calories:* ~33
- *Carbs:* 6g
- *Fiber:* 1g

8. Zucchini:
Serving: **1 medium zucchini**
- *Calories:* ~33
- *Carbs:* 6g
- *Fiber:* 2g

9. Brussels Sprouts:
Serving: **1 cup (cooked)**
- *Calories:* ~56
- *Carbs:* 12g
- *Fiber:* 4g

10. Cauliflower:
Serving: **1 cup (chopped)**

- *Calories:* ~27
- *Carbs:* 5g
- *Fiber:* 2g

11. Asparagus:
Serving: 1 cup (cooked)
- *Calories:* ~27
- *Carbs:* 5g
- *Fiber:* 3g

12. Green Beans:
Serving: 1 cup (cooked)
- *Calories:* ~44
- *Carbs:* 10g
- *Fiber:* 4g

13. Sweet Potatoes:
Serving: 1 medium sweet potato
- *Calories:* ~103
- *Carbs:* 24g
- *Fiber:* 4g

14. Onions:
Serving: **1 medium onion**
- *Calories:* ~44
- *Carbs:* 10g
- *Fiber:* 2g

15. Garlic:
Serving: **1 clove**
- *Calories:* ~4
- *Carbs:* 1g
- *Fiber:* 0.1g

16. Mushrooms:
Serving: **1 cup (sliced)**
- *Calories:* ~15
- *Carbs:* 3g
- *Fiber:* 1g

17. Cabbage:
Serving: **1 cup (shredded)**
- *Calories:* ~22
- *Carbs:* 5g

- *Fiber:* 2g

18. Eggplant:
***Serving:* 1 cup (cubed)**
- *Calories:* ~20
- *Carbs:* 5g
- *Fiber:* 3g

19. Artichokes:
***Serving:* 1 medium artichoke**
- *Calories:* ~60
- *Carbs:* 13g
- *Fiber:* 7g

20. Butternut Squash:
***Serving:* 1 cup (cubed)**
- *Calories:* ~82
- *Carbs:* 22g
- *Fiber:* 7g

PLANT-BASED PROTEINS

1. Lentils:
- *Protein:* ~18g per cup (cooked)

2. Chickpeas:
- *Protein:* ~15g per cup (cooked)

3. Black Beans:
- *Protein:* ~15g per cup (cooked)

4. Quinoa:
- *Protein:* ~8g per cup (cooked)

5. Tofu:

Protein: ~20g per cup (firm, raw)

6. Tempeh:
- *Protein:* ~31g per cup (cooked)

7. Edamame:
- *Protein:* ~17g per cup (cooked)

8. Hemp Seeds:
- *Protein:* ~10g per 3 tablespoons (hulled)

9. Chia Seeds:
- *Protein:* ~4g per 2 tablespoons (dried)

10. Almonds:
- *Protein:* ~6g per 1/4 cup (dry roasted)

11. Peanuts:

Protein: ~9g per 1/4 cup (dry roasted)

12. Sunflower Seeds:
- *Protein:* ~6g per 1/4 cup (dry roasted)

13. Buckwheat:
- *Protein:* ~6g per cup (cooked)

14. Brown Rice:
- *Protein:* ~5g per cup (cooked)

15. Seitan:
- *Protein:* ~21g per 3 ounces (cooked)

16. Soy Milk:
- *Protein:* ~8g per cup

17. Spinach:
- *Protein:* ~5g per cup (cooked)

18. Broccoli:
- *Protein:* ~3g per cup (cooked)

19. Brussels Sprouts:
- *Protein:* ~3g per cup (cooked)

20. Spirulina:
- *Protein:* ~4g per tablespoon (dried)

- **FATTY FISH**

1. Salmon:

Serving: **3 ounces**

- *Calories:* ~206
- *Protein:* 22g
- *Omega-3s:* 1,828mg

2. Mackerel:

Serving: **3 ounces**

- *Calories:* ~330
- *Protein:* 31g
- *Omega-3s:* 4,580mg

3. Sardines:

Serving: **3 ounces**

- *Calories:* ~191

- *Protein:* 22g
- *Omega-3s:* 1,480mg

4. Trout:
***Serving:* 3 ounces**

- *Calories:* ~148
- *Protein:* 21g
- *Omega-3s:* 1,035mg

5. Herring:
***Serving:* 3 ounces**

- *Calories:* ~200
- *Protein:* 18g
- *Omega-3s:* 1,710mg

6. Anchovies:
***Serving:* 2 ounces (canned)**

- *Calories:* ~94
- *Protein:* 13g
- *Omega-3s:* 952mg

7. Albacore Tuna:
Serving: **3 ounces**
- *Calories:* ~109
- *Protein:* 20g
- *Omega-3s:* 823mg

8. Rainbow Trout:
Serving: **3 ounces**
- *Calories:* ~144
- *Protein:* 18g
- *Omega-3s:* 1,088mg

9. Halibut:
Serving: **3 ounces**
- *Calories:* ~94
- *Protein:* 20g
- *Omega-3s:* 490mg

10. Arctic Char:
Serving: **3 ounces**
- *Calories:* ~153
- *Protein:* 19g

- *Omega-3s:* 1,000mg

11. Barramundi:
Serving: **3 ounces**
- *Calories:* ~90
- *Protein:* 18g
- *Omega-3s:* 400mg

12. Black Cod (Sablefish):
Serving: **3 ounces**
- *Calories:* ~200
- *Protein:* 16g
- *Omega-3s:* 1,480mg

13. Bluefish:
Serving: **3 ounces**
- *Calories:* ~175
- *Protein:* 20g
- *Omega-3s:* 1,800mg

14. Cobia:
Serving: **3 ounces**

- *Calories:* ~87
- *Protein:* 17g
- *Omega-3s:* 272mg

15. Mahi-Mahi:
Serving: **3 ounces**
- *Calories:* ~85
- *Protein:* 18g
- *Omega-3s:* 150mg

16. Whitefish:
Serving: **3 ounces**
- *Calories:* ~105
- *Protein:* 20g
- *Omega-3s:* 1,000mg

17. Canned Mackerel:
Serving: **3 ounces (canned)**
- *Calories:* ~230
- *Protein:* 22g
- *Omega-3s:* 4,580mg

18. Spanish Mackerel:

Serving: **3 ounces**

- *Calories:* ~230
- *Protein:* 22g
- *Omega-3s:* 3,000mg

19. Striped Bass:

Serving: **3 ounces**

- *Calories:* ~105
- *Protein:* 19g
- *Omega-3s:* 495mg

20. Alaskan Pollock:

Serving: **3 ounces**

- *Calories:* ~80
- *Protein:* 19g
- *Omega-3s:* 470mg

- **WHOLE GRAINS**

1. Quinoa:

Serving: 1 cup, cooked

- *Calories:* ~222
- *Carbs:* 39g
- *Fiber:* 5.2g

2. Brown Rice:

Serving: 1 cup, cooked

- *Calories:* ~218
- *Carbs:* 45g
- *Fiber:* 3.5g

3. Oats:

Serving: 1 cup, cooked

- *Calories:* ~147
- *Carbs:* 25g
- *Fiber:* 4g

4. Barley:

Serving: 1 cup, cooked

- *Calories:* ~193

- *Carbs:* 44g
- *Fiber:* 6g

5. Farro:
***Serving:* 1 cup, cooked**
- *Calories:* ~220
- *Carbs:* 47g
- *Fiber:* 9g

6. Bulgur:
***Serving:* 1 cup, cooked**
- *Calories:* ~151
- *Carbs:* 34g
- *Fiber:* 8g

7. Millet:
***Serving:* 1 cup, cooked**
- *Calories:* ~207
- *Carbs:* 41g
- *Fiber:* 2.3g

8. Whole Wheat Pasta:
Serving: 1 cup, cooked
- *Calories:* ~174
- *Carbs:* 37g
- *Fiber:* 6g

9. Freekeh:
Serving: 1 cup, cooked
- *Calories:* ~240
- *Carbs:* 46g
- *Fiber:* 12g

10. Buckwheat:
Serving: 1 cup, cooked
- *Calories:* ~155
- *Carbs:* 33g
- *Fiber:* 5.8g

11. Sorghum:
Serving: 1 cup, cooked
- *Calories:* ~651
- *Carbs:* 143g

- *Fiber:* 12g

12. Wild Rice:
***Serving:* 1 cup, cooked**
- *Calories:* ~166
- *Carbs:* 35g
- *Fiber:* 3g

13. Amaranth:
***Serving:* 1 cup, cooked**
- *Calories:* ~251
- *Carbs:* 46g
- *Fiber:* 5.2g

14. Teff:
***Serving:* 1 cup, cooked**
- *Calories:* ~255
- *Carbs:* 50g
- *Fiber:* 10g

15. Spelt:
Serving: **1 cup, cooked**
- *Calories:* ~246
- *Carbs:* 51g
- *Fiber:* 7.6g

16. Kamut:
Serving: **1 cup, cooked**
- *Calories:* ~227
- *Carbs:* 48g
- *Fiber:* 7g

17. Soba Noodles (Buckwheat):
Serving: **1 cup, cooked**
- *Calories:* ~113
- *Carbs:* 25g
- *Fiber:* 3g

18. Einkorn Wheat:
Serving: **1 cup, cooked**
- *Calories:* ~184
- *Carbs:* 38g

- *Fiber:* 5g

19. Rye:
Serving: **1 cup, cooked**
- *Calories:* ~176
- *Carbs:* 37g
- *Fiber:* 14g

20. Black Rice (Forbidden Rice):
Serving: **1 cup, cooked**
- *Calories:* ~160
- *Carbs:* 35g
- *Fiber:* 3g

- **LEAFY GREENS:**

1. Spinach:
Serving: **1 cup, raw**
- *Calories:* ~7
- *Carbs:* 1g
- *Fiber:* 0.7g

2. Kale:
Serving: 1 cup, raw

- *Calories:* ~33
- *Carbs:* 6g
- *Fiber:* 1.3g

3. Swiss Chard:
Serving: 1 cup, raw

- *Calories:* ~7
- *Carbs:* 1.4g
- *Fiber:* 0.6g

4. Collard Greens:
Serving: 1 cup, cooked

- *Calories:* ~63
- *Carbs:* 11g
- *Fiber:* 8g

5. Arugula:
Serving: 1 cup, raw

- *Calories:* ~5
- *Carbs:* 0.5g

- *Fiber:* 0.3g

6. Romaine Lettuce:

Serving: **1 cup, shredded**

- *Calories:* ~8
- *Carbs:* 1.5g
- *Fiber:* 1g

7. Cabbage (Green):

Serving: **1 cup, shredded**

- *Calories:* ~22
- *Carbs:* 5g
- *Fiber:* 2.2g

8. Bok Choy:

Serving: **1 cup, shredded**

- *Calories:* ~9
- *Carbs:* 1.5g
- *Fiber:* 0.7g

9. Iceberg Lettuce:

Serving: **1 cup, shredded**

- *Calories:* ~10
- *Carbs:* 2g
- *Fiber:* 1g

10. Beet Greens:

Serving: **1 cup, cooked**

- *Calories:* ~39
- *Carbs:* 8g
- *Fiber:* 4g

11. Turnip Greens:

Serving: **1 cup, cooked**

- *Calories:* ~29
- *Carbs:* 6g
- *Fiber:* 4g

12. Mustard Greens:

Serving: **1 cup, cooked**

- *Calories:* ~21
- *Carbs:* 4g
- *Fiber:* 3g

13. Watercress:
Serving: 1 cup, raw
- *Calories:* ~4
- *Carbs:* 0.4g
- *Fiber:* 0.2g

14. Endive:
Serving: 1 cup, raw
- *Calories:* ~8
- *Carbs:* 1.7g
- *Fiber:* 1.6g

15. Chicory Greens:
Serving: 1 cup, raw
- *Calories:* ~23
- *Carbs:* 5g
- *Fiber:* 2.5g

HERBS & SPICES

1. Turmeric:
Amount: 1 teaspoon, ground

- *Calories:* ~9
- *Carbs:* 2g
- *Fiber:* 1g

2. Ginger:
Amount: 1 tablespoon, grated
- *Calories:* ~5
- *Carbs:* 1g
- *Fiber:* 0g

3. Cinnamon:
Amount: 1 teaspoon, ground
- *Calories:* ~6
- *Carbs:* 2g
- *Fiber:* 1g

4. Garlic:
Amount: 1 clove, minced
- *Calories:* ~4
- *Carbs:* 1g
- *Fiber:* 0g

5. Basil:

Amount: 1 tablespoon, fresh

- *Calories:* ~1
- *Carbs:* 0g
- *Fiber:* 0g

6. Oregano:

Amount: 1 teaspoon, dried

- *Calories:* ~3
- *Carbs:* 1g
- *Fiber:* 1g

7. Rosemary:

Amount: 1 tablespoon, fresh

- *Calories:* ~2
- *Carbs:* 0g
- *Fiber:* 0g

8. Thyme:

Amount: 1 teaspoon, dried

- *Calories:* ~3

- *Carbs:* 1g
- *Fiber:* 0g

9. Cayenne Pepper:

Amount: **1 teaspoon, ground**

- *Calories:* ~6
- *Carbs:* 1g
- *Fiber:* 1g

10. Parsley:

Amount: **1 tablespoon, fresh**

- *Calories:* ~1
- *Carbs:* 0g
- *Fiber:* 0g

11. Mint:

Amount: **1 tablespoon, fresh**

- *Calories:* ~1
- *Carbs:* 0g
- *Fiber:* 0g

12. Coriander (Cilantro):
Amount: **1 tablespoon, fresh**

- *Calories:* ~0
- *Carbs:* 0g
- *Fiber:* 0g

13. Sage:
Amount: **1 teaspoon, ground**

- *Calories:* ~6
- *Carbs:* 1g
- *Fiber:* 1g

14. Dill:
Amount: **1 tablespoon, fresh**

- *Calories:* ~1
- *Carbs:* 0g
- *Fiber:* 0g

15. Fennel Seeds:
Amount: **1 teaspoon, whole**

- *Calories:* ~6

- *Carbs:* 1g
- *Fiber:* 1g

16. Turmeric:
Amount: **1 teaspoon, ground**

- *Calories:* ~9
- *Carbs:* 2g
- *Fiber:* 1g

17. Black Pepper:
Amount: **1 teaspoon, ground**

- *Calories:* ~6
- *Carbs:* 1g
- *Fiber:* 0g

18. Cloves:
Amount: **1 teaspoon, ground**

- *Calories:* ~6
- *Carbs:* 1g
- *Fiber:* 1g

19. Chives:

Amount: **1 tablespoon, fresh**

- *Calories:* ~1
- *Carbs:* 0g
- *Fiber:* 0g

20. Cumin:

Amount: **1 teaspoon, ground**

- *Calories:* ~8
- *Carbs:* 1g
- *Fiber:* 0g

- **NUTS & SEEDS**

1. Almonds:

Amount: **1 ounce (about 23 almonds)**

- *Calories:* ~160
- *Carbs:* 6g
- *Fiber:* 3.5g

2. Walnuts:
Amount: 1 ounce (about 14 halves)
- *Calories:* ~185
- *Carbs:* 4g
- *Fiber:* 2g

3. Flaxseeds:
Amount: 1 tablespoon, ground
- *Calories:* ~37
- *Carbs:* 2g
- *Fiber:* 1.9g

4. Chia Seeds:
Amount: 1 ounce (about 2 tablespoons)
- *Calories:* ~138
- *Carbs:* 12g
- *Fiber:* 9.8g

5. Pumpkin Seeds (Pepitas):
Amount: 1 ounce (about 85 seeds)
- *Calories:* ~151
- *Carbs:* 5g

- *Fiber:* 1.1g

6. Sunflower Seeds:
Amount: **1 ounce (about 87 seeds)**
- *Calories:* ~204
- *Carbs:* 7g
- *Fiber:* 3.5g

7. Brazil Nuts:
Amount: **1 ounce (about 6 nuts)**
- *Calories:* ~186
- *Carbs:* 3g
- *Fiber:* 2.1g

8. Pistachios:
Amount: **1 ounce (about 49 kernels)**
- *Calories:* ~159
- *Carbs:* 8g
- *Fiber:* 3g

9. Cashews:
Amount: **1 ounce (about 18 nuts)**

- *Calories:* ~155
- *Carbs:* 9g
- *Fiber:* 1g

10. Hemp Seeds:

Amount: **1 ounce (about 3 tablespoons)**

- *Calories:* ~166
- *Carbs:* 3g
- *Fiber:* 1.2g

11. Sesame Seeds:

Amount: **1 tablespoon**

- *Calories:* ~52
- *Carbs:* 4g
- *Fiber:* 1.9g

12. Pecans:

Amount: **1 ounce (about 19 halves)**

- *Calories:* ~196
- *Carbs:* 4g
- *Fiber:* 2.7g

13. Macadamia Nuts:

Amount: **1 ounce (about 10–12 nuts)**

- *Calories:* ~204
- *Carbs:* 4g
- *Fiber:* 2.4g

14. Hazelnuts (Filberts):

Amount: **1 ounce (about 21 nuts)**

- *Calories:* ~176
- *Carbs:* 5g
- *Fiber:* 3g

15. Chia Seeds:

Amount: **1 ounce (about 2 tablespoons)**

- *Calories:* ~138
- *Carbs:* 12g
- *Fiber:* 9.8g

- **FOODS FILLED WITH OMEGA-3 FATTY ACIDS**

1. Salmon:

Serving: **3 ounces, cooked**

- *Calories:* ~175
- *Omega-3s (EPA/DHA):* ~1,000mg

2. Chia Seeds:

Serving: **1 ounce**

- *Calories:* ~138
- *Omega-3s (ALA):* ~4,915mg

3. Walnuts:

Serving: **1 ounce**

- *Calories:* ~185
- *Omega-3s (ALA):* ~2,570mg

4. Flaxseeds:

Serving: **1 tablespoon, ground**

- *Calories:* ~37
- *Omega-3s (ALA):* ~2,350mg

5. Sardines:

Serving: **3.2 ounces, canned in oil**
- *Calories:* ~190
- *Omega-3s (EPA/DHA):* ~1,480mg

6. Hemp Seeds:

Serving: **1 ounce**
- *Calories:* ~155
- *Omega-3s (ALA):* ~1,000mg

7. Mackerel:

Serving: **3 ounces, cooked**
- *Calories:* ~230
- *Omega-3s (EPA/DHA):* ~4,580mg

8. Algal Oil (Plant-Based Omega-3 Supplement):

Serving: **1 capsule (usually 300-600mg DHA)**
- *Calories:* Varies

9. Edamame:

Serving: **1 cup, cooked**

- *Calories:* ~189
- *Omega-3s (ALA):* ~670mg

10. Brussels Sprouts:
Serving: 1 cup, cooked
- *Calories:* ~56
- *Omega-3s (ALA):* ~260mg

11. Krill Oil:
Serving: 1 capsule (usually 60-120mg EPA/DHA)
- *Calories:* Varies

12. Seaweed (Nori):
Serving: 1 sheet
- *Calories:* ~10
- *Omega-3s (ALA):* ~60mg

13. Tofu:
Serving: 4 ounces, raw
- *Calories:* ~94
- *Omega-3s (ALA):* ~280mg

14. Scallops:
Serving: **3 ounces, cooked**
- *Calories:* ~95
- *Omega-3s (EPA/DHA):* ~350mg

15. Cauliflower:
Serving: **1 cup, raw**
- *Calories:* ~27
- *Omega-3s (ALA):* ~80mg

16. Grass-Fed Beef:
Serving: **3 ounces, cooked**
- *Calories:* ~180
- *Omega-3s (ALA):* ~30mg

17. Herring:
Serving: **3 ounces, cooked**
- *Calories:* ~210
- *Omega-3s (EPA/DHA):* ~1,300mg

18. Eggs (Enriched with Omega-3):
Serving: **1 large egg**
- *Calories:* ~70
- *Omega-3s (ALA):* ~75mg

19. Shrimp:
Serving: **3 ounces, cooked**
- *Calories:* ~84
- *Omega-3s (EPA/DHA):* ~270mg

20. Soybean Oil:
Serving: **1 tablespoon**
- *Calories:* ~120
- *Omega-3s (ALA):* ~930mg

- **COFFEE**

1. Black Coffee:
Amount: **1 cup**
- *Calories:* ~2
- *Carbs:* 0g
- *Fiber:* 0g

2. Turmeric Latte (Golden Milk Coffee):

Amount: 1 cup

- *Calories:* ~50
- *Carbs:* 8g
- *Fiber:* 1g

3. Cinnamon Coffee:

Amount: 1 cup

- *Calories:* ~2
- *Carbs:* 0.6g
- *Fiber:* 0.4g

4. Gingerbread Coffee:

Amount: 1 cup

- *Calories:* ~5
- *Carbs:* 1g
- *Fiber:* 0g

5. Coconut Oil Coffee (Bulletproof Coffee):

Amount: 1 cup

- *Calories:* ~120
- *Carbs:* 0g
- *Fiber:* 0g

6. Mint Mocha:

***Amount:* 1 cup**
- *Calories:* ~40
- *Carbs:* 8g
- *Fiber:* 1g

7. Cocoa Cinnamon Coffee:
***Amount:* 1 cup**
- *Calories:* ~5
- *Carbs:* 1g
- *Fiber:* 0.7g

8. Vanilla Almond Coffee:
***Amount:* 1 cup**
- *Calories:* ~20
- *Carbs:* 2g
- *Fiber:* 0.5g

9. Chai Spiced Coffee:
***Amount:* 1 cup**
- *Calories:* ~5
- *Carbs:* 1g
- *Fiber:* 0g

10. Hibiscus Cold Brew:

Amount: **1 cup**

- *Calories:* ~5
- *Carbs:* 1g
- *Fiber:* 0g

- **GREEN TEA**

1. Matcha Green Tea:

Amount: **1 teaspoon, powdered**

- *Calories:* ~3
- *Carbs:* 0.6g
- *Fiber:* 0.4g

2. Sencha Green Tea:

Amount: **1 teaspoon, loose leaves**

- *Calories:* ~0
- *Carbs:* 0g
- *Fiber:* 0g

3. Gunpowder Green Tea:

Amount: **1 teaspoon, loose leaves**

- *Calories:* ~0

- *Carbs:* 0g
- *Fiber:* 0g

4. Jasmine Green Tea:

Amount: 1 teaspoon, loose leaves

- *Calories:* ~0
- *Carbs:* 0g
- *Fiber:* 0g

5. Dragon Well (Longjing) Green Tea:

Amount: 1 teaspoon, loose leaves

- *Calories:* ~0
- *Carbs:* 0g
- *Fiber:* 0g

6. Genmaicha Green Tea:

Amount: 1 teaspoon, loose leaves

- *Calories:* ~0
- *Carbs:* 0g
- *Fiber:* 0g

7. Hojicha Green Tea:

Amount: 1 teaspoon, loose leaves

- *Calories:* ~0

- *Carbs:* 0g
- *Fiber:* 0g

8. Bancha Green Tea:
Amount: 1 teaspoon, loose leaves

- *Calories:* ~0
- *Carbs:* 0g
- *Fiber:* 0g

9. Kukicha Green Tea:
Amount: 1 teaspoon, loose leaves

- *Calories:* ~0
- *Carbs:* 0g
- *Fiber:* 0g

10. Moroccan Mint Green Tea:
Amount: 1 teaspoon, loose leaves

- *Calories:* ~0
- *Carbs:* 0g
- *Fiber:* 0g

DARK CHOCOLATE (IN MODERATION)

1. 70% Dark Chocolate:

***Amount:* 1 ounce**

- *Calories:* ~170
- *Carbs:* 13g
- *Fiber:* 3g

2. 85% Dark Chocolate:

***Amount:* 1 ounce**

- *Calories:* ~170
- *Carbs:* 12g
- *Fiber:* 3g

3. 90% Dark Chocolate:

***Amount:* 1 ounce**

- *Calories:* ~150
- *Carbs:* 9g
- *Fiber:* 3g

4. 95% Dark Chocolate:

***Amount:* 1 ounce**

- *Calories:* ~170
- *Carbs:* 6g

- *Fiber:* 3g

5. Dark Chocolate Covered Almonds:

***Amount:* 1 ounce**

- *Calories:* ~160
- *Carbs:* 10g
- *Fiber:* 3g

6. Dark Chocolate with Sea Salt:

***Amount:* 1 ounce**

- *Calories:* ~150
- *Carbs:* 12g
- *Fiber:* 2g

7. Dark Chocolate with Almonds and Cranberries:

***Amount:* 1 ounce**

- *Calories:* ~140
- *Carbs:* 12g
- *Fiber:* 3g

8. Dark Chocolate with Ginger:

***Amount:* 1 ounce**

- *Calories:* ~160
- *Carbs:* 13g
- *Fiber:* 2g

9. Dark Chocolate with Mint:
Amount: **1 ounce**
- *Calories:* ~150
- *Carbs:* 11g
- *Fiber:* 3g

10. Dark Chocolate with Pomegranate:
Amount: **1 ounce**
- *Calories:* ~160
- *Carbs:* 16g
- *Fiber:* 3g

Remember to enjoy dark chocolate in moderation as part of a balanced diet. The higher the cocoa content, the better, as it tends to have more anti-inflammatory properties.

RED WINE (IN MODERATION)

1. Cabernet Sauvignon:
Amount: **5 fluid ounces**
- *Calories:* ~123
- *Carbs:* 3.9g
- *Sugar:* 0.6g

2. Merlot:

Amount: **5 fluid ounces**

- *Calories:* ~122
- *Carbs:* 3.7g
- *Sugar:* 0.6g

3. Pinot Noir:

Amount: **5 fluid ounces**

- *Calories:* ~121
- *Carbs:* 3.4g
- *Sugar:* 0.4g

4. Syrah/Shiraz:

Amount: **5 fluid ounces**

- *Calories:* ~122
- *Carbs:* 3.79g
- *Sugar:* 0.55g

5. Malbec:

Amount: **5 fluid ounces**

- *Calories:* ~122
- *Carbs:* 3.8g
- *Sugar:* 0.47g

6. Zinfandel:

Amount: **5 fluid ounces**
- *Calories:* ~129
- *Carbs:* 4.2g
- *Sugar:* 1g

7. Tempranillo:

Amount: **5 fluid ounces**
- *Calories:* ~122
- *Carbs:* 3.9g
- *Sugar:* 0.5g

8. Barbera:

Amount: **5 fluid ounces**
- *Calories:* ~131
- *Carbs:* 4.3g
- *Sugar:* 0.3g

9. Grenache:

Amount: **5 fluid ounces**
- *Calories:* ~122
- *Carbs:* 3.8g
- *Sugar:* 0.4g

10. Sangiovese:

Amount: **5 fluid ounces**
- *Calories:* ~126

- *Carbs:* 3.9g
- *Sugar:* 0.5g

11.   Châteauneuf-du-Pape:

Amount: **5 fluid ounces**

- *Calories:* ~127
- *Carbs:* 3.4g
- *Sugar:* 0.5g

12.   Petite Sirah:

Amount: **5 fluid ounces**

- *Calories:* ~132
- *Carbs:* 4g
- *Sugar:* 0.7g

13.   Côtes du Rhône:

Amount: **5 fluid ounces**

- *Calories:* ~130
- *Carbs:* 3.8g
- *Sugar:* 0.6g

14.   Cabernet Franc:

Amount: **5 fluid ounces**

- *Calories:* ~123
- *Carbs:* 3.9g
- *Sugar:* 0.6g

15. Mourvèdre:

Amount: **5 fluid ounces**

- *Calories:* ~132
- *Carbs:* 4g
- *Sugar:* 0.5g

Remember to enjoy these in moderation as part of a balanced and healthy diet. Cheers!

ANTI INFLAMMATORY DIET MEAL PLANNING TIPS:

An anti-inflammatory diet can be a transformative journey for your health. By focusing on foods known for their anti-inflammatory properties, you pave the way for improved well-being. Here are 15 practical meal planning tips to guide your dietary choices and support your journey towards a more inflammation-friendly lifestyle.

- **Colorful Veggies:** Include a variety of colorful vegetables for diverse nutrients and antioxidants.
- **Omega-3s:** Incorporate fatty fish, flaxseeds, and chia seeds for anti-inflammatory omega-3 fatty acids.
- **Whole Grains:** Choose whole grains like quinoa and oats for fiber and anti-inflammatory benefits.
- **Healthy Fats:** Opt for olive oil, avocados, and nuts for heart-healthy fats.
- **Lean Proteins:** Include lean sources like chicken, beans, and tofu to support muscle health.
- **Herbs & Spices:** Use turmeric, ginger, and garlic for natural anti-inflammatory properties.

- **Limit Processed Foods:** Minimize processed items for a cleaner, inflammation-friendly diet.
- **Hydration:** Stay well-hydrated with water and herbal teas to support your overall health.
- **Colorful Plate:** Aim for a variety of colors on your plate to ensure diverse nutrient intake.
- **Moderate Alcohol:** If consumed, opt for moderate amounts, particularly red wine for antioxidants.
- **Mindful Eating:** Practice mindful eating to savor meals and control portion sizes.
- **Limit Added Sugars:** Reduce added sugars; get sweetness from natural sources like fruits.
- **Fiber-Rich Choices:** Choose high-fiber foods like legumes and whole grains for gut health.
- **Probiotics:** Incorporate yogurt or kefir for gut-friendly probiotics.
- **Consult a Professional:** Seek guidance from a nutritionist or healthcare professional for personalized advice.

QUICK AND EASY ANTI-INFLAMMATORY DELICIOUS RECIPES

BREAKFAST

1. Avocado and Salmon Breakfast Wrap:

- **Ingredients:** Whole-grain wrap, smoked salmon, avocado, cherry tomatoes, spinach.
- **Directions:** Spread mashed avocado on the wrap, layer with salmon, tomatoes, and spinach. Roll it up and enjoy.

2. Berry and Almond Smoothie Bowl:

- **Ingredients:** Mixed berries, banana, almond milk, chia seeds, almonds.
- **Directions:** Blend berries, banana, and almond milk; pour into a bowl. Top with chia seeds and almonds.

3. Turmeric Scrambled Eggs:

- **Ingredients:** Eggs, turmeric, spinach, cherry tomatoes, olive oil.

- **Directions:** Scramble eggs with turmeric, sauté spinach and tomatoes in olive oil, combine.

4. Greek Yogurt Parfait with Nuts:

- **Ingredients:** Greek yogurt, mixed nuts, honey, blueberries.
- **Directions:** Layer Greek yogurt with nuts and blueberries, drizzle with honey.

5. Quinoa Breakfast Bowl:

- **Ingredients:** Quinoa, coconut milk, mango, kiwi, shredded coconut.
- **Directions:** Cook quinoa in coconut milk, top with sliced mango, kiwi, and shredded coconut.

LUNCH

1. Grilled Chicken and Vegetable Salad:

- **Ingredients:** Grilled chicken breast, mixed greens, cherry tomatoes, cucumber, bell peppers, olive oil.
- **Directions:** Toss grilled chicken and veggies over mixed greens, drizzle with olive oil.

2. Quinoa and Black Bean Bowl:

- **Ingredients:** Quinoa, black beans, corn, avocado, lime, cilantro.
- **Directions:** Mix cooked quinoa, black beans, corn; top with sliced avocado, lime juice, and cilantro.

3. Salmon and Sweet Potato Skewers:

- **Ingredients:** Salmon cubes, sweet potato chunks, olive oil, lemon, rosemary.
- **Directions:** Skewer salmon and sweet potato, brush with olive oil, bake until cooked, garnish with lemon and rosemary.

4. Lentil and Vegetable Soup:

- **Ingredients:** Lentils, carrots, celery, onion, garlic, vegetable broth, turmeric.
- **Directions:** Sauté veggies, add lentils, broth, and turmeric; simmer until lentils are tender.

5. Spinach and Chickpea Salad:

- **Ingredients:** Fresh spinach, chickpeas, cherry tomatoes, feta cheese, balsamic vinaigrette.
- **Directions:** Combine spinach, chickpeas, tomatoes, and feta; drizzle with balsamic vinaigrette.

DINNER:

1. Baked Turmeric Cod with Quinoa:

- **Ingredients:** Cod fillets, turmeric, lemon, quinoa, broccoli.
- **Directions:** Season cod with turmeric and lemon, bake. Serve over quinoa with steamed broccoli.

2. Vegetable Stir-Fry with Tofu:

- **Ingredients:** Tofu, mixed vegetables (broccoli, bell peppers, snap peas), ginger, soy sauce.
- **Directions:** Sauté tofu and veggies with ginger and soy sauce until cooked.

3. Butternut Squash and Chickpea Curry:

- **Ingredients:** Butternut squash, chickpeas, coconut milk, curry spices, brown rice.
- **Directions:** Cook butternut squash and chickpeas in coconut milk with curry spices. Serve over brown rice.

4. Turkey and Quinoa Stuffed Bell Peppers:

- **Ingredients:** Ground turkey, quinoa, bell peppers, tomatoes, black beans.
- **Directions:** Cook turkey and quinoa, mix with tomatoes and black beans. Stuff bell peppers, bake until tender.

5. Sweet Potato and Kale Hash:

- **Ingredients:** Sweet potatoes, kale, onion, garlic, olive oil, poached egg.
- **Directions:** Sauté sweet potatoes, kale, onion, and garlic in olive oil. Top with a poached egg.

SNACKS

1. Greek Yogurt with Berries:

- **Ingredients:** Greek yogurt, mixed berries, honey.
- **Directions:** Top Greek yogurt with mixed berries and drizzle with honey.

2. Almond Butter and Banana Slices:

- **Ingredients:** Whole-grain rice cakes, almond butter, banana.
- **Directions:** Spread almond butter on rice cakes, top with banana slices.

3. Hummus and Veggie Sticks:

- **Ingredients:** Hummus, carrot sticks, cucumber slices and bell pepper strips.
- **Directions:** Dip veggie sticks into hummus for a satisfying snack.

4. Trail Mix with Nuts and Seeds:

- **Ingredients:** Mixed nuts, seeds, dried fruits.

- **Directions:** Create a custom trail mix with your favorite nuts, seeds, and dried fruits.

5. Avocado and Tomato on Whole Grain Toast:

- **Ingredients:** Whole-grain bread, avocado, tomato slices, sea salt.
- **Directions:** Spread mashed avocado on toast, top with tomato slices, sprinkle with sea salt.

DESSERTS

1. Chia Seed Pudding with Berries:

- **Ingredients:** Chia seeds, almond milk, mixed berries, vanilla extract.
- **Directions:** Mix the chia seeds with almond milk and vanilla extract. Refrigerate, then top with mixed berries.

2. Baked Apples with Cinnamon and Walnuts:

- **Ingredients:** Apples, cinnamon, walnuts, honey.
- **Directions:** Core apples, fill with walnuts and cinnamon, bake until tender. Drizzle with honey.

3. Dark Chocolate and Berry Parfait:

- **Ingredients:** Dark chocolate, Greek yogurt, mixed berries.
- **Directions:** Layer melted dark chocolate, Greek yogurt, and mixed berries in a parfait glass.

4. Mango and Coconut Sorbet:

- **Ingredients:** Frozen mango chunks, coconut milk, lime juice.
- **Directions:** Blend frozen mango, coconut milk, and lime juice until smooth. Freeze until desired consistency.

5. Almond Flour Banana Muffins:

- **Ingredients:** Almond flour, ripe bananas, eggs, baking soda.
- **Directions:** Mix almond flour, mashed bananas, eggs, and baking soda. Bake into muffins.

SMOOTHIES

1. Green Detox Smoothie:

- **Ingredients:** Spinach, cucumber, green apple, lemon, ginger, water.
- **Directions:** Blend spinach, cucumber, apple, lemon, and ginger with water.

2. Berry Protein Smoothie:

- **Ingredients:** Mixed berries, protein powder, almond milk, chia seeds.
- **Directions:** Blend berries, protein powder, almond milk, and chia seeds until smooth.

3. Tropical Turmeric Smoothie:

- **Ingredients:** Pineapple, mango, turmeric, coconut water.
- **Directions:** Blend pineapple, mango, turmeric, and coconut water for a refreshing drink.

4. Avocado and Kale Smoothie:

- **Ingredients:** Avocado, kale, banana, Greek yogurt, almond milk.
- **Directions:** Blend avocado, kale, banana, Greek yogurt, and almond milk until creamy.

5. Chocolate Peanut Butter Banana Smoothie:

- **Ingredients:** Banana, cocoa powder, peanut butter, almond milk.
- **Directions:** Blend banana, cocoa powder, peanut butter, and almond milk for a chocolatey treat.

Enjoy these Anti-inflammatory recipes, rich in nutrients and flavor. Adjust ingredients to suit your taste preferences and dietary requirements.

BUILDING A HEART-HEALTHY FRIENDLY PANTRY: ESSENTIAL GROCERY LIST

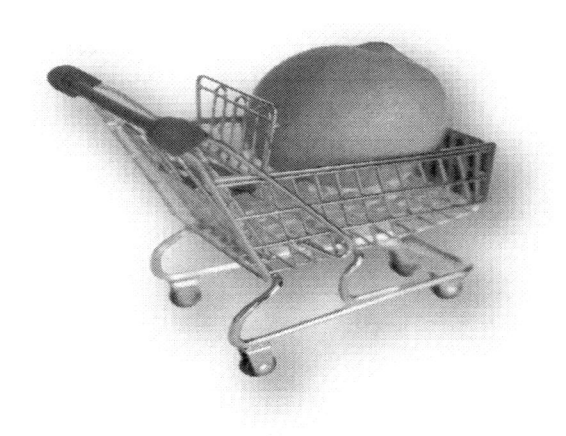

BREAKFAST

1. *Avocado and Salmon Breakfast Wrap:*

- Whole-grain wraps
- Smoked salmon
- Avocado
- Cherry tomatoes
- Spinach

2. Berry and Almond Smoothie Bowl:

- Mixed berries (fresh or frozen)
- Banana
- Almond milk
- Chia seeds
- Almonds

3. Turmeric Scrambled Eggs:

- Eggs
- Turmeric
- Spinach
- Cherry tomatoes
- Olive oil

4. Greek Yogurt Parfait with Nuts:

- Greek yogurt
- Mixed nuts
- Honey
- Blueberries

5. Quinoa Breakfast Bowl:

- Quinoa
- Coconut milk
- Mango

- Kiwi
- Shredded coconut

LUNCH

1. *Grilled Chicken and Vegetable Salad:*

- Grilled chicken breast
- Mixed greens
- Cherry tomatoes
- Cucumber
- Bell peppers
- Olive oil

2. *Quinoa and Black Bean Bowl:*

- Quinoa
- Black beans
- Corn
- Avocado
- Lime
- Cilantro

3. *Salmon and Sweet Potato Skewers:*

- Salmon fillets
- Sweet potatoes

- Olive oil
- Lemon
- Fresh rosemary

4. Lentil and Vegetable Soup:

- Lentils
- Carrots
- Celery
- Onion
- Garlic
- Vegetable broth
- Turmeric

5. Spinach and Chickpea Salad:

- Fresh spinach
- Chickpeas
- Cherry tomatoes
- Feta cheese
- Balsamic vinaigrette

DINNER

1. Baked Turmeric Cod with Quinoa:

- Cod fillets

- Turmeric
- Lemon
- Quinoa
- Broccoli

2. *Vegetable Stir-Fry with Tofu:*

- Tofu
- Mixed vegetables (broccoli, bell peppers, snap peas)
- Ginger
- Soy sauce

3. *Butternut Squash and Chickpea Curry:*

- Butternut squash
- Chickpeas
- Coconut milk
- Curry spices
- Brown rice

4. *Turkey and Quinoa Stuffed Bell Peppers:*

- Ground turkey
- Quinoa
- Bell peppers
- Tomatoes
- Black beans

5. Sweet Potato and Kale Hash:

- Sweet potatoes
- Kale
- Onion
- Garlic
- Olive oil
- Eggs (for poaching)

SNACKS

1. Greek Yogurt with Berries:

- Greek yogurt
- Mixed berries
- Honey

2. Almond Butter and Banana Slices:

- Whole-grain rice cakes
- Almond butter
- Banana

3. Hummus and Veggie Sticks:

- Hummus
- Carrot sticks
- Cucumber slices

- Bell pepper strips

4. *Trail Mix with Nuts and Seeds:*

- Mixed nuts
- Seeds
- Dried fruits

5. *Avocado and Tomato on Whole Grain Toast:*

- Whole-grain bread
- Avocado
- Tomato slices
- Sea salt

DESSERTS

1. Chia Seed Pudding with Berries:

- Chia seeds
- Almond milk
- Mixed berries
- Vanilla extract

2. *Baked Apples with Cinnamon and Walnuts:*

- Apples
- Cinnamon
- Walnuts

- Honey

3. *Dark Chocolate and Berry Parfait:*

- Dark chocolate
- Greek yogurt
- Mixed berries

4. *Mango and Coconut Sorbet:*

- Frozen mango chunks
- Coconut milk
- Lime juice

5. *Almond Flour Banana Muffins:*

- Almond flour
- Ripe bananas
- Eggs
- Baking soda

SMOOTHIES

1. *Green Detox Smoothie:*

- Spinach
- Cucumber
- Green apple
- Lemon

- Ginger
- Water

2. *Berry Protein Smoothie:*

- Mixed berries (fresh or frozen)
- Protein powder
- Almond milk
- Chia seeds

3. *Tropical Turmeric Smoothie:*

- Pineapple
- Mango
- Turmeric
- Coconut water

4. *Avocado and Kale Smoothie:*

- Avocado
- Kale
- Banana
- Greek yogurt
- Almond milk

5. *Chocolate Peanut Butter Banana Smoothie:*

- Banana
- Cocoa powder

- Peanut butter
- Almond milk

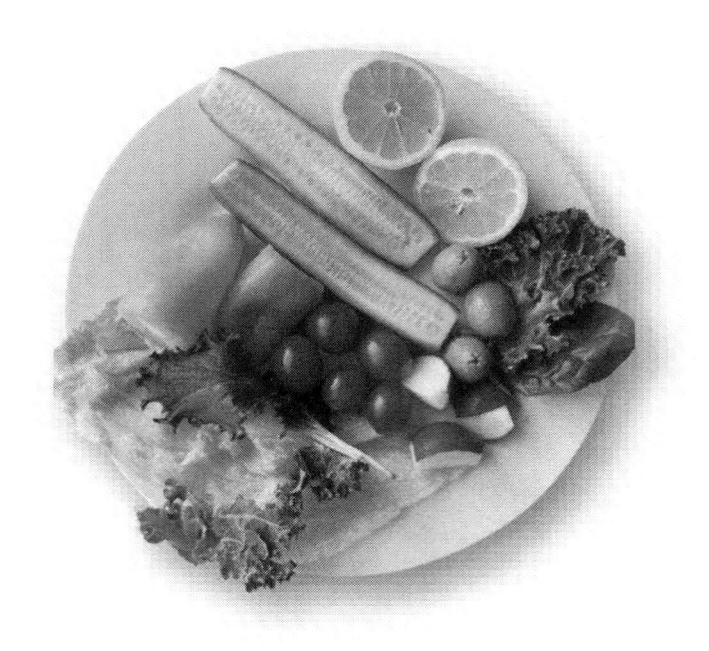

Feel free to adjust quantities based on your preferences and household size. Happy cooking

CONCLUSION

Adopting an anti-inflammatory diet is a holistic approach to promoting overall health and well-being. The foods outlined in the chart offer a diverse array of nutrient-rich options that not only combat inflammation but also contribute to a balanced and satisfying culinary experience.

By incorporating these choices into your daily meals, you are not just nourishing your body but actively supporting its natural defense mechanisms.

The chart emphasizes the importance of whole foods, rich in antioxidants, omega-3 fatty acids, and a variety of vitamins and minerals. These components collectively work to reduce inflammation, mitigate oxidative stress, and support optimal bodily functions.

The versatility of the recommended ingredients allows for creativity in meal planning, ensuring that maintaining an anti-inflammatory diet doesn't become monotonous.

Moreover, the variety of recipes provided caters to different tastes and preferences, making the transition to an anti-inflammatory lifestyle accessible and enjoyable. Whether it's a nutrient-packed smoothie for breakfast, a vibrant salad for lunch, or a flavorful curry for dinner, each recipe is designed to be not only health-conscious but also delicious.

Incorporating these dietary choices is a positive step toward fostering a healthier relationship with food and establishing long-term habits that prioritize well-being. Remember, small changes can lead to significant improvements in how your body feels and functions, contributing to a more vibrant and energetic life.

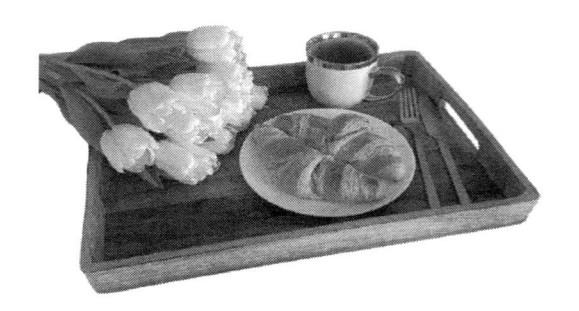

HAPPY COOKING!

Printed in Dunstable, United Kingdom